SHIFT RESET JOURNAL

A GUIDED RESET FOR LIFE ON THE CLOCK

For permission requests, contact:

Birds of a Feather Consulting Group, Inc.
birdsoffeatherconsulting@gmail.com
www.myERnurse.com
Imacel ·Cel· Robinson, BSN RN

Disclaimer:
This journal is intended for personal reflection and wellness support.
It does not constitute medical advice, diagnosis, or treatment.
Always seek guidance from a licensed medical professional for any
health concerns.

WELCOME TO THE SHIFT RESET JOURNAL

Long shifts. Heavy hearts. Full schedules.

In the world of healthcare, it's easy to care for everyone else and forget to check in with yourself. This journal was created as a space for you — the caregiver, the responder, the one who keeps going. Whether you're on day shift, night shift, or in between, these pages are here to help you pause, process, and reset.

WHAT YOU'LL FIND INSIDE:

• 90 daily journaling pages with reflection prompts
• Motivational quotes and wellness reminders
• Space to acknowledge the emotional, mental, and physical weight of your shift
• A final page to reflect on your journey

HOW TO USE IT:

There's no wrong way to show up here. Write what you feel.
Skip a day if you need. Revisit moments that mattered.

Let this journal meet you where you are.
You don't have to pour from an empty cup.

This is your space to refill — one shift at a time.
Imacel ·Cel· Robinson, BSN RN

@officiallookitscelly

All quotes in this journal are original reflections crafted for this publication

DAY 1

What's something that challenged you today?

_____

_____

_____

_____

_____

What's something that gave you joy or purpose?

_____

_____

_____

_____

_____

How did your body feel after today's shift?

_____

_____

_____

_____

_____

What's one thing you want to reset or release?

_____

_____

_____

_____

_____

How can you support yourself before your next shift?

_____

_____

_____

_____

_____

You showed up. That counts for something.

DAY 2

What's something that challenged you today?

_____
_____
_____
_____
_____

What's something that gave you joy or purpose?

_____
_____
_____
_____
_____

How did your body feel after today's shift?

_____
_____
_____
_____
_____

What's one thing you want to reset or release?

_____
_____
_____
_____
_____

How can you support yourself before your next shift?

_____
_____
_____
_____
_____

Not every day has to be your best day. Today was enough.

DAY 3

What's something that challenged you today?

_____

_____

_____

_____

_____

What's something that gave you joy or purpose?

_____

_____

_____

_____

How did your body feel after today's shift?

_____

_____

_____

_____

What's one thing you want to reset or release?

_____

_____

_____

_____

How can you support yourself before your next shift?

_____

_____

_____

_____

_____

Drink water. You're not just tired -- you might be dehydrated.

DAY 4

What's something that challenged you today?

_____

_____

_____

_____

_____

What's something that gave you joy or purpose?

_____

_____

_____

_____

_____

How did your body feel after today's shift?

_____

_____

_____

_____

_____

What's one thing you want to reset or release?

_____

_____

_____

_____

_____

How can you support yourself before your next shift?

_____

_____

_____

_____

_____

Healing doesn't always look heroic. Sometimes it's just being kind to yourself.

DAY 5

What's something that challenged you today?

_____

_____

_____

_____

_____

What's something that gave you joy or purpose?

_____

_____

_____

_____

_____

How did your body feel after today's shift?

_____

_____

_____

_____

_____

What's one thing you want to reset or release?

_____

_____

_____

_____

_____

How can you support yourself before your next shift?

_____

_____

_____

_____

_____

You don't have to explain your exhaustion. Your shift explains it for you.

DAY 6

What's something that challenged you today?

_____

_____

_____

_____

_____

What's something that gave you joy or purpose?

_____

_____

_____

_____

_____

How did your body feel after today's shift?

_____

_____

_____

_____

_____

What's one thing you want to reset or release?

_____

_____

_____

_____

_____

How can you support yourself before your next shift?

_____

_____

_____

_____

_____

No one can pour from an empty cup. Please refill yours.

DAY 7

What's something that challenged you today?

_____

_____

_____

_____

_____

What's something that gave you joy or purpose?

_____

_____

_____

_____

_____

How did your body feel after today's shift?

_____

_____

_____

_____

_____

What's one thing you want to reset or release?

_____

_____

_____

_____

_____

How can you support yourself before your next shift?

_____

_____

_____

_____

_____

That thing you're beating yourself up about' You handled it better than you think.

DAY 8

What's something that challenged you today?

_____

_____

_____

_____

_____

What's something that gave you joy or purpose?

_____

_____

_____

_____

_____

How did your body feel after today's shift?

_____

_____

_____

_____

_____

What's one thing you want to reset or release?

_____

_____

_____

_____

_____

How can you support yourself before your next shift?

_____

_____

_____

_____

_____

Stretch your back, unclench your jaw, and give yourself some credit.

DAY 9

What's something that challenged you today?

_____

_____

_____

_____

_____

What's something that gave you joy or purpose?

_____

_____

_____

_____

_____

How did your body feel after today's shift?

_____

_____

_____

_____

_____

What's one thing you want to reset or release?

_____

_____

_____

_____

_____

How can you support yourself before your next shift?

_____

_____

_____

_____

_____

Feeling numb doesn't mean you don't care -- it means you've cared too much for too long.

DAY 10

What's something that challenged you today?

_____

_____

_____

_____

_____

What's something that gave you joy or purpose?

_____

_____

_____

_____

_____

How did your body feel after today's shift?

_____

_____

_____

_____

_____

What's one thing you want to reset or release?

_____

_____

_____

_____

_____

How can you support yourself before your next shift?

_____

_____

_____

_____

_____

A reset isn't selfish. It's survival.

DAY 11

What's something that challenged you today?

_____

_____

_____

_____

_____

What's something that gave you joy or purpose?

_____

_____

_____

_____

_____

How did your body feel after today's shift?

_____

_____

_____

_____

_____

What's one thing you want to reset or release?

_____

_____

_____

_____

_____

How can you support yourself before your next shift?

_____

_____

_____

_____

_____

You don't owe anyone perfection -- just presence.

DAY 12

What's something that challenged you today?

_____

_____

_____

_____

_____

What's something that gave you joy or purpose?

_____

_____

_____

_____

How did your body feel after today's shift?

_____

_____

_____

_____

What's one thing you want to reset or release?

_____

_____

_____

_____

How can you support yourself before your next shift?

_____

_____

_____

_____

Close your eyes for 60 seconds. Breathe like it matters. Because it does.

DAY 13

What's something that challenged you today?

_____
_____
_____
_____
_____

What's something that gave you joy or purpose?

_____
_____
_____
_____
_____

How did your body feel after today's shift?

_____
_____
_____
_____

What's one thing you want to reset or release?

_____
_____
_____
_____

How can you support yourself before your next shift?

_____
_____
_____
_____

Hard shifts are part of the job. But they're not your whole story.

DAY 14

What's something that challenged you today?

_____
_____
_____
_____
_____

What's something that gave you joy or purpose?

_____
_____
_____
_____
_____

How did your body feel after today's shift?

_____
_____
_____
_____
_____

What's one thing you want to reset or release?

_____
_____
_____
_____
_____

How can you support yourself before your next shift?

_____
_____
_____
_____
_____

You're allowed to have limits -- even if you're
the strong one.

DAY 15

What's something that challenged you today?

_____

_____

_____

_____

_____

What's something that gave you joy or purpose?

_____

_____

_____

_____

_____

How did your body feel after today's shift?

_____

_____

_____

_____

_____

What's one thing you want to reset or release?

_____

_____

_____

_____

_____

How can you support yourself before your next shift?

_____

_____

_____

_____

_____

This is a reminder to eat something real -- not just caffeine and graham crackers.

DAY 16

What's something that challenged you today?

_____

_____

_____

_____

_____

What's something that gave you joy or purpose?

_____

_____

_____

_____

_____

How did your body feel after today's shift?

_____

_____

_____

_____

_____

What's one thing you want to reset or release?

_____

_____

_____

_____

_____

How can you support yourself before your next shift?

_____

_____

_____

_____

_____

You were the calm in someone's chaos today. That matters.

DAY 17

What's something that challenged you today?

_____

_____

_____

_____

_____

What's something that gave you joy or purpose?

_____

_____

_____

_____

_____

How did your body feel after today's shift?

_____

_____

_____

_____

_____

What's one thing you want to reset or release?

_____

_____

_____

_____

_____

How can you support yourself before your next shift?

_____

_____

_____

_____

_____

Grace is giving yourself the compassion you give everyone else.

DAY 18

What's something that challenged you today?

_____

_____

_____

_____

_____

What's something that gave you joy or purpose?

_____

_____

_____

_____

_____

How did your body feel after today's shift?

_____

_____

_____

_____

_____

What's one thing you want to reset or release?

_____

_____

_____

_____

_____

How can you support yourself before your next shift?

_____

_____

_____

_____

_____

Sleep is a form of therapy. Give yourself a full session.

DAY 19

What's something that challenged you today?

_____
_____
_____
_____
_____

What's something that gave you joy or purpose?

_____
_____
_____
_____
_____

How did your body feel after today's shift?

_____
_____
_____
_____
_____

What's one thing you want to reset or release?

_____
_____
_____
_____
_____

How can you support yourself before your next shift?

_____
_____
_____
_____
_____

It's okay to care deeply and still need distance.
That's not weakness -- that's wisdom.

DAY 20

What's something that challenged you today?

_____
_____
_____
_____
_____

What's something that gave you joy or purpose?

_____
_____
_____
_____
_____

How did your body feel after today's shift?

_____
_____
_____
_____
_____

What's one thing you want to reset or release?

_____
_____
_____
_____
_____

How can you support yourself before your next shift?

_____
_____
_____
_____
_____

You've already done more than most people could handle. That's strength.

DAY 21

What's something that challenged you today?

_____

_____

_____

_____

_____

What's something that gave you joy or purpose?

_____

_____

_____

_____

_____

How did your body feel after today's shift?

_____

_____

_____

_____

_____

What's one thing you want to reset or release?

_____

_____

_____

_____

_____

How can you support yourself before your next shift?

_____

_____

_____

_____

_____

Wipe the day off your skin -- literally. A hot shower resets more than just muscles.

DAY 22

What's something that challenged you today?

_____

_____

_____

_____

_____

What's something that gave you joy or purpose?

_____

_____

_____

_____

_____

How did your body feel after today's shift?

_____

_____

_____

_____

_____

What's one thing you want to reset or release?

_____

_____

_____

_____

_____

How can you support yourself before your next shift?

_____

_____

_____

_____

_____

You don't have to bounce back. You can take your time.

DAY 23

What's something that challenged you today?

_____

_____

_____

_____

_____

What's something that gave you joy or purpose?

_____

_____

_____

_____

_____

How did your body feel after today's shift?

_____

_____

_____

_____

_____

What's one thing you want to reset or release?

_____

_____

_____

_____

_____

How can you support yourself before your next shift?

_____

_____

_____

_____

_____

Name one thing you're proud of. Now say it out loud.

DAY 24

What's something that challenged you today?

_____

_____

_____

_____

_____

What's something that gave you joy or purpose?

_____

_____

_____

_____

_____

How did your body feel after today's shift?

_____

_____

_____

_____

_____

What's one thing you want to reset or release?

_____

_____

_____

_____

_____

How can you support yourself before your next shift?

_____

_____

_____

_____

_____

Nothing resets like a moment of stillness. One breath. One pause.

DAY 25

What's something that challenged you today?

_____

_____

_____

_____

_____

What's something that gave you joy or purpose?

_____

_____

_____

_____

_____

How did your body feel after today's shift?

_____

_____

_____

_____

_____

What's one thing you want to reset or release?

_____

_____

_____

_____

_____

How can you support yourself before your next shift?

_____

_____

_____

_____

_____

Your badge isn't your identity. You are more than your role.

DAY 26

What's something that challenged you today?

_____
_____
_____
_____
_____

What's something that gave you joy or purpose?

_____
_____
_____
_____
_____

How did your body feel after today's shift?

_____
_____
_____
_____
_____

What's one thing you want to reset or release?

_____
_____
_____
_____
_____

How can you support yourself before your next shift?

_____
_____
_____
_____

Headphones in. World off. Protect your peace.

DAY 27

What's something that challenged you today?

_____
_____
_____
_____
_____

What's something that gave you joy or purpose?

_____
_____
_____
_____
_____

How did your body feel after today's shift?

_____
_____
_____
_____
_____

What's one thing you want to reset or release?

_____
_____
_____
_____
_____

How can you support yourself before your next shift?

_____
_____
_____
_____

You can do brave things gently.

DAY 28

What's something that challenged you today?

_____
_____
_____
_____
_____

What's something that gave you joy or purpose?

_____
_____
_____
_____
_____

How did your body feel after today's shift?

_____
_____
_____
_____
_____

What's one thing you want to reset or release?

_____
_____
_____
_____
_____

How can you support yourself before your next shift?

_____
_____
_____
_____

Set a boundary. Keep it. Protect your damn energy.

DAY 29

What's something that challenged you today?

_____

_____

_____

_____

_____

What's something that gave you joy or purpose?

_____

_____

_____

_____

_____

How did your body feel after today's shift?

_____

_____

_____

_____

_____

What's one thing you want to reset or release?

_____

_____

_____

_____

_____

How can you support yourself before your next shift?

_____

_____

_____

_____

_____

Reclaim five minutes for yourself. No guilt. No apology.

DAY 30

What's something that challenged you today?

_____

_____

_____

_____

_____

What's something that gave you joy or purpose?

_____

_____

_____

_____

_____

How did your body feel after today's shift?

_____

_____

_____

_____

_____

What's one thing you want to reset or release?

_____

_____

_____

_____

_____

How can you support yourself before your next shift?

_____

_____

_____

_____

_____

Reminder: You're not alone in this. Even when it feels like it.

DAY 31

What's something that challenged you today?

_____
_____
_____
_____
_____

What's something that gave you joy or purpose?

_____
_____
_____
_____
_____

How did your body feel after today's shift?

_____
_____
_____
_____
_____

What's one thing you want to reset or release?

_____
_____
_____
_____
_____

How can you support yourself before your next shift?

_____
_____
_____
_____
_____

Your best today might look different than
yesterday. That's okay.

DAY 32

What's something that challenged you today?

_____

_____

_____

_____

_____

What's something that gave you joy or purpose?

_____

_____

_____

_____

_____

How did your body feel after today's shift?

_____

_____

_____

_____

_____

What's one thing you want to reset or release?

_____

_____

_____

_____

How can you support yourself before your next shift?

_____

_____

_____

_____

Look away from the screen for 20 seconds. Your
eyes deserve a reset too.

DAY 33

What's something that challenged you today?

_____

_____

_____

_____

_____

What's something that gave you joy or purpose?

_____

_____

_____

_____

How did your body feel after today's shift?

_____

_____

_____

_____

What's one thing you want to reset or release?

_____

_____

_____

_____

How can you support yourself before your next shift?

_____

_____

_____

_____

_____

You're allowed to exhale. No one expects you to carry it all.

DAY 34

What's something that challenged you today?

_____

_____

_____

_____

_____

What's something that gave you joy or purpose?

_____

_____

_____

_____

_____

How did your body feel after today's shift?

_____

_____

_____

_____

_____

What's one thing you want to reset or release?

_____

_____

_____

_____

_____

How can you support yourself before your next shift?

_____

_____

_____

_____

_____

Use the cool compress. Your eyes have seen enough for one day.

DAY 35

What's something that challenged you today?

_____

_____

_____

_____

_____

What's something that gave you joy or purpose?

_____

_____

_____

_____

_____

How did your body feel after today's shift?

_____

_____

_____

_____

_____

What's one thing you want to reset or release?

_____

_____

_____

_____

_____

How can you support yourself before your next shift?

_____

_____

_____

_____

_____

You didn't just survive that shift. You softened chaos. That's a superpower.

DAY 36

What's something that challenged you today?

_____

_____

_____

_____

_____

What's something that gave you joy or purpose?

_____

_____

_____

_____

_____

How did your body feel after today's shift?

_____

_____

_____

_____

_____

What's one thing you want to reset or release?

_____

_____

_____

_____

_____

How can you support yourself before your next shift?

_____

_____

_____

_____

_____

Blue light isn't just annoying -- it's exhausting.
Rest your eyes in the dark for a few minutes.

DAY 37

What's something that challenged you today?

_____
_____
_____
_____
_____

What's something that gave you joy or purpose?

_____
_____
_____
_____
_____

How did your body feel after today's shift?

_____
_____
_____
_____
_____

What's one thing you want to reset or release?

_____
_____
_____
_____
_____

How can you support yourself before your next shift?

_____
_____
_____
_____

You don't have to hold everything together for everyone. You're someone too.

DAY 38

What's something that challenged you today?

_____
_____
_____
_____
_____

What's something that gave you joy or purpose?

_____
_____
_____
_____
_____

How did your body feel after today's shift?

_____
_____
_____
_____
_____

What's one thing you want to reset or release?

_____
_____
_____
_____
_____

How can you support yourself before your next shift?

_____
_____
_____
_____
_____

Warm your hands and rest them gently over your eyes. Close. Breathe.

DAY 39

What's something that challenged you today?

_____

_____

_____

_____

_____

What's something that gave you joy or purpose?

_____

_____

_____

_____

_____

How did your body feel after today's shift?

_____

_____

_____

_____

_____

What's one thing you want to reset or release?

_____

_____

_____

_____

_____

How can you support yourself before your next shift?

_____

_____

_____

_____

_____

There's strength in staying soft. Let gentleness be your rebellion.

DAY 40

What's something that challenged you today?

_____

_____

_____

_____

_____

What's something that gave you joy or purpose?

_____

_____

_____

_____

_____

How did your body feel after today's shift?

_____

_____

_____

_____

_____

What's one thing you want to reset or release?

_____

_____

_____

_____

_____

How can you support yourself before your next shift?

_____

_____

_____

_____

_____

If your eyes sting, that's not weakness -- it's a
cry for rest. Listen.

DAY 41

What's something that challenged you today?

_____

_____

_____

_____

_____

What's something that gave you joy or purpose?

_____

_____

_____

_____

_____

How did your body feel after today's shift?

_____

_____

_____

_____

_____

What's one thing you want to reset or release?

_____

_____

_____

_____

_____

How can you support yourself before your next shift?

_____

_____

_____

_____

_____

You don't have to keep showing up at 100%. Showing up is enough.

DAY 42

What's something that challenged you today?

_____

_____

_____

_____

_____

What's something that gave you joy or purpose?

_____

_____

_____

_____

_____

How did your body feel after today's shift?

_____

_____

_____

_____

_____

What's one thing you want to reset or release?

_____

_____

_____

_____

_____

How can you support yourself before your next shift?

_____

_____

_____

_____

_____

Your vision blurs because you've been focusing on everyone else all day. Look inward now.

DAY 43

What's something that challenged you today?

_____

_____

_____

_____

_____

What's something that gave you joy or purpose?

_____

_____

_____

_____

_____

How did your body feel after today's shift?

_____

_____

_____

_____

_____

What's one thing you want to reset or release?

_____

_____

_____

_____

_____

How can you support yourself before your next shift?

_____

_____

_____

_____

_____

Just because you handled it all doesn't mean it was easy. Let yourself feel it.

DAY 44

What's something that challenged you today?

_____

_____

_____

_____

_____

What's something that gave you joy or purpose?

_____

_____

_____

_____

_____

How did your body feel after today's shift?

_____

_____

_____

_____

_____

What's one thing you want to reset or release?

_____

_____

_____

_____

_____

How can you support yourself before your next shift?

_____

_____

_____

_____

_____

Cool cloth. Quiet room. Eyes closed. You deserve 10 uninterrupted minutes.

DAY 45

What's something that challenged you today?

_____

_____

_____

_____

_____

What's something that gave you joy or purpose?

_____

_____

_____

_____

_____

How did your body feel after today's shift?

_____

_____

_____

_____

_____

What's one thing you want to reset or release?

_____

_____

_____

_____

_____

How can you support yourself before your next shift?

_____

_____

_____

_____

_____

You weren't meant to run on empty. Power down. Literally.

DAY 46

What's something that challenged you today?

_____
_____
_____
_____
_____

What's something that gave you joy or purpose?

_____
_____
_____
_____
_____

How did your body feel after today's shift?

_____
_____
_____
_____
_____

What's one thing you want to reset or release?

_____
_____
_____
_____
_____

How can you support yourself before your next shift?

_____
_____
_____
_____
_____

Let your tears flow. That's not weakness -- that's biology.

DAY 47

What's something that challenged you today?

_____

_____

_____

_____

_____

What's something that gave you joy or purpose?

_____

_____

_____

_____

_____

How did your body feel after today's shift?

_____

_____

_____

_____

_____

What's one thing you want to reset or release?

_____

_____

_____

_____

_____

How can you support yourself before your next shift?

_____

_____

_____

_____

_____

That chart can wait. Your corneas can't. Blink.
Breathe. Break.

DAY 48

What's something that challenged you today?

_____

_____

_____

_____

_____

What's something that gave you joy or purpose?

_____

_____

_____

_____

_____

How did your body feel after today's shift?

_____

_____

_____

_____

_____

What's one thing you want to reset or release?

_____

_____

_____

_____

_____

How can you support yourself before your next shift?

_____

_____

_____

_____

Healing work takes a toll on healers too. Step back and recalibrate.

DAY 49

What's something that challenged you today?

_____

_____

_____

_____

_____

What's something that gave you joy or purpose?

_____

_____

_____

_____

How did your body feel after today's shift?

_____

_____

_____

_____

What's one thing you want to reset or release?

_____

_____

_____

_____

How can you support yourself before your next shift?

_____

_____

_____

_____

_____

Protect your peace like your paycheck. It's just as valuable.

DAY 50

What's something that challenged you today?

_____

_____

_____

_____

_____

What's something that gave you joy or purpose?

_____

_____

_____

_____

_____

How did your body feel after today's shift?

_____

_____

_____

_____

_____

What's one thing you want to reset or release?

_____

_____

_____

_____

_____

How can you support yourself before your next shift?

_____

_____

_____

_____

_____

Soft light. Eye drops. No scrolling. Give your eyes a screen detox.

DAY 51

What's something that challenged you today?

_____

_____

_____

_____

_____

What's something that gave you joy or purpose?

_____

_____

_____

_____

How did your body feel after today's shift?

_____

_____

_____

_____

What's one thing you want to reset or release?

_____

_____

_____

_____

How can you support yourself before your next shift?

_____

_____

_____

_____

This weight you're carrying' You're allowed to set it down.

DAY 52

What's something that challenged you today?

_____

_____

_____

_____

_____

What's something that gave you joy or purpose?

_____

_____

_____

_____

_____

How did your body feel after today's shift?

_____

_____

_____

_____

_____

What's one thing you want to reset or release?

_____

_____

_____

_____

_____

How can you support yourself before your next shift?

_____

_____

_____

_____

_____

Close your eyes and visualize peace. A few seconds is still self-care.

DAY 53

What's something that challenged you today?

_____

_____

_____

_____

_____

What's something that gave you joy or purpose?

_____

_____

_____

_____

_____

How did your body feel after today's shift?

_____

_____

_____

_____

_____

What's one thing you want to reset or release?

_____

_____

_____

_____

_____

How can you support yourself before your next shift?

_____

_____

_____

_____

_____

Dry eyes' Blurred vision' That's your body whispering, "Slow down."

DAY 54

What's something that challenged you today?

_____

_____

_____

_____

_____

What's something that gave you joy or purpose?

_____

_____

_____

_____

_____

How did your body feel after today's shift?

_____

_____

_____

_____

What's one thing you want to reset or release?

_____

_____

_____

_____

How can you support yourself before your next shift?

_____

_____

_____

_____

_____

You made decisions, helped strangers, and still remembered your own name. That's badass.

DAY 55

What's something that challenged you today?

_____

_____

_____

_____

_____

What's something that gave you joy or purpose?

_____

_____

_____

_____

_____

How did your body feel after today's shift?

_____

_____

_____

_____

What's one thing you want to reset or release?

_____

_____

_____

_____

How can you support yourself before your next shift?

_____

_____

_____

_____

_____

The Shift Reset Journal is your permission slip to pause.

DAY 56

What's something that challenged you today?

_____

_____

_____

_____

_____

What's something that gave you joy or purpose?

_____

_____

_____

_____

_____

How did your body feel after today's shift?

_____

_____

_____

_____

_____

What's one thing you want to reset or release?

_____

_____

_____

_____

_____

How can you support yourself before your next shift?

_____

_____

_____

_____

_____

Your mind is overstimulated. Your eyes are overworked. You are overdue for rest.

DAY 57

What's something that challenged you today?

_____

_____

_____

_____

_____

What's something that gave you joy or purpose?

_____

_____

_____

_____

_____

How did your body feel after today's shift?

_____

_____

_____

_____

_____

What's one thing you want to reset or release?

_____

_____

_____

_____

_____

How can you support yourself before your next shift?

_____

_____

_____

_____

_____

Boundaries are the bravest form of self-respect.
Keep holding them.

DAY 58

What's something that challenged you today?

_____
_____
_____
_____
_____

What's something that gave you joy or purpose?

_____
_____
_____
_____
_____

How did your body feel after today's shift?

_____
_____
_____
_____
_____

What's one thing you want to reset or release?

_____
_____
_____
_____
_____

How can you support yourself before your next shift?

_____
_____
_____
_____
_____

Dim the lights. Rub your temples. Breathe like your nervous system matters.

DAY 59

What's something that challenged you today?

_____

_____

_____

_____

_____

What's something that gave you joy or purpose?

_____

_____

_____

_____

_____

How did your body feel after today's shift?

_____

_____

_____

_____

_____

What's one thing you want to reset or release?

_____

_____

_____

_____

_____

How can you support yourself before your next shift?

_____

_____

_____

_____

_____

Try the 20-20-20 rule: every 20 minutes, look 20 feet away for 20 seconds.

DAY 60

What's something that challenged you today?

_____

_____

_____

_____

_____

What's something that gave you joy or purpose?

_____

_____

_____

_____

_____

How did your body feel after today's shift?

_____

_____

_____

_____

_____

What's one thing you want to reset or release?

_____

_____

_____

_____

_____

How can you support yourself before your next shift?

_____

_____

_____

_____

_____

There is no trophy for overextending. You're allowed to rest -- deeply.

DAY 61

What's something that challenged you today?

_____

_____

_____

_____

_____

What's something that gave you joy or purpose?

_____

_____

_____

_____

_____

How did your body feel after today's shift?

_____

_____

_____

_____

_____

What's one thing you want to reset or release?

_____

_____

_____

_____

_____

How can you support yourself before your next shift?

_____

_____

_____

_____

_____

You deserve hydration that isn't half coffee.

DAY 62

What's something that challenged you today?

_____

_____

_____

_____

_____

What's something that gave you joy or purpose?

_____

_____

_____

_____

_____

How did your body feel after today's shift?

_____

_____

_____

_____

_____

What's one thing you want to reset or release?

_____

_____

_____

_____

_____

How can you support yourself before your next shift?

_____

_____

_____

_____

_____

Close your eyes for one minute. Let the world wait.

DAY 63

What's something that challenged you today?

_____

_____

_____

_____

_____

What's something that gave you joy or purpose?

_____

_____

_____

_____

_____

How did your body feel after today's shift?

_____

_____

_____

_____

_____

What's one thing you want to reset or release?

_____

_____

_____

_____

_____

How can you support yourself before your next shift?

_____

_____

_____

_____

_____

You were not built to go full throttle forever.
Slow is not failure.

DAY 64

What's something that challenged you today?

_____

_____

_____

_____

_____

What's something that gave you joy or purpose?

_____

_____

_____

_____

_____

How did your body feel after today's shift?

_____

_____

_____

_____

_____

What's one thing you want to reset or release?

_____

_____

_____

_____

_____

How can you support yourself before your next shift?

_____

_____

_____

_____

_____

Warm lemon water. Deep breath. Keep it simple today.

DAY 65

What's something that challenged you today?

_____

_____

_____

_____

_____

What's something that gave you joy or purpose?

_____

_____

_____

_____

_____

How did your body feel after today's shift?

_____

_____

_____

_____

_____

What's one thing you want to reset or release?

_____

_____

_____

_____

_____

How can you support yourself before your next shift?

_____

_____

_____

_____

_____

That aching head' Could be dehydration. Could be stress. Could be both. Start with water.

DAY 66

What's something that challenged you today?

_____

_____

_____

_____

_____

What's something that gave you joy or purpose?

_____

_____

_____

_____

_____

How did your body feel after today's shift?

_____

_____

_____

_____

_____

What's one thing you want to reset or release?

_____

_____

_____

_____

_____

How can you support yourself before your next shift?

_____

_____

_____

_____

_____

If you're not sleeping, you're not healing. Power down early tonight.

DAY 67

What's something that challenged you today?

_____

_____

_____

_____

_____

What's something that gave you joy or purpose?

_____

_____

_____

_____

_____

How did your body feel after today's shift?

_____

_____

_____

_____

_____

What's one thing you want to reset or release?

_____

_____

_____

_____

_____

How can you support yourself before your next shift?

_____

_____

_____

_____

_____

You've been strong all day. It's okay to fall apart now.

DAY 68

What's something that challenged you today?

_____

_____

_____

_____

_____

What's something that gave you joy or purpose?

_____

_____

_____

_____

How did your body feel after today's shift?

_____

_____

_____

_____

What's one thing you want to reset or release?

_____

_____

_____

_____

How can you support yourself before your next shift?

_____

_____

_____

_____

Your body isn't an inconvenience -- it's your home. Care for it like it matters.

DAY 69

What's something that challenged you today?

_____

_____

_____

_____

_____

What's something that gave you joy or purpose?

_____

_____

_____

_____

_____

How did your body feel after today's shift?

_____

_____

_____

_____

_____

What's one thing you want to reset or release?

_____

_____

_____

_____

_____

How can you support yourself before your next shift?

_____

_____

_____

_____

_____

No one thrives off crumbs. Eat something real.
You're not too busy to be nourished.

DAY 70

What's something that challenged you today?

_____

_____

_____

_____

_____

What's something that gave you joy or purpose?

_____

_____

_____

_____

_____

How did your body feel after today's shift?

_____

_____

_____

_____

_____

What's one thing you want to reset or release?

_____

_____

_____

_____

_____

How can you support yourself before your next shift?

_____

_____

_____

_____

Stretch. Hydrate. Let your muscles know you still live here.

DAY 71

What's something that challenged you today?

_____

_____

_____

_____

_____

What's something that gave you joy or purpose?

_____

_____

_____

_____

_____

How did your body feel after today's shift?

_____

_____

_____

_____

_____

What's one thing you want to reset or release?

_____

_____

_____

_____

_____

How can you support yourself before your next shift?

_____

_____

_____

_____

_____

Breathe into your belly. The kind of breath that signals safety.

DAY 72

What's something that challenged you today?

_____

_____

_____

_____

_____

What's something that gave you joy or purpose?

_____

_____

_____

_____

How did your body feel after today's shift?

_____

_____

_____

_____

What's one thing you want to reset or release?

_____

_____

_____

_____

How can you support yourself before your next shift?

_____

_____

_____

_____

_____

Sip slowly. You're not rushing a code. You're tending to yourself.

DAY 73

What's something that challenged you today?

_____

_____

_____

_____

_____

What's something that gave you joy or purpose?

_____

_____

_____

_____

_____

How did your body feel after today's shift?

_____

_____

_____

_____

_____

What's one thing you want to reset or release?

_____

_____

_____

_____

_____

How can you support yourself before your next shift?

_____

_____

_____

_____

_____

Sleep is not optional. It's sacred.

DAY 74

What's something that challenged you today?

_____
_____
_____
_____
_____

What's something that gave you joy or purpose?

_____
_____
_____
_____

How did your body feel after today's shift?

_____
_____
_____
_____

What's one thing you want to reset or release?

_____
_____
_____
_____

How can you support yourself before your next shift?

_____
_____
_____
_____

You are not required to be reachable at all hours.
Protect your peace.

DAY 75

What's something that challenged you today?

_____

_____

_____

_____

_____

What's something that gave you joy or purpose?

_____

_____

_____

_____

_____

How did your body feel after today's shift?

_____

_____

_____

_____

_____

What's one thing you want to reset or release?

_____

_____

_____

_____

_____

How can you support yourself before your next shift?

_____

_____

_____

_____

_____

Eyes closed. Palms open. Say nothing. Just be.

DAY 76

What's something that challenged you today?

_____

_____

_____

_____

_____

What's something that gave you joy or purpose?

_____

_____

_____

_____

_____

How did your body feel after today's shift?

_____

_____

_____

_____

_____

What's one thing you want to reset or release?

_____

_____

_____

_____

_____

How can you support yourself before your next shift?

_____

_____

_____

_____

_____

Soft food. Soft lighting. Soft thoughts. Your nervous system is begging for gentle.

DAY 77

What's something that challenged you today?

_____

_____

_____

_____

_____

What's something that gave you joy or purpose?

_____

_____

_____

_____

_____

How did your body feel after today's shift?

_____

_____

_____

_____

_____

What's one thing you want to reset or release?

_____

_____

_____

_____

_____

How can you support yourself before your next shift?

_____

_____

_____

_____

_____

What if today, "doing your best" meant listening to your body'

DAY 78

What's something that challenged you today?

_____

_____

_____

_____

_____

What's something that gave you joy or purpose?

_____

_____

_____

_____

_____

How did your body feel after today's shift?

_____

_____

_____

_____

_____

What's one thing you want to reset or release?

_____

_____

_____

_____

_____

How can you support yourself before your next shift?

_____

_____

_____

_____

_____

Hydrate before you caffeinate. Your organs will thank you.

DAY 79

What's something that challenged you today?

_____

_____

_____

_____

_____

What's something that gave you joy or purpose?

_____

_____

_____

_____

_____

How did your body feel after today's shift?

_____

_____

_____

_____

_____

What's one thing you want to reset or release?

_____

_____

_____

_____

_____

How can you support yourself before your next shift?

_____

_____

_____

_____

_____

There is nothing noble about burnout.

DAY 80

What's something that challenged you today?

_____

_____

_____

_____

_____

What's something that gave you joy or purpose?

_____

_____

_____

_____

_____

How did your body feel after today's shift?

_____

_____

_____

_____

_____

What's one thing you want to reset or release?

_____

_____

_____

_____

_____

How can you support yourself before your next shift?

_____

_____

_____

_____

_____

Just because you're good at functioning in chaos doesn't mean you should have to.

DAY 81

What's something that challenged you today?

_____
_____
_____
_____
_____

What's something that gave you joy or purpose?

_____
_____
_____
_____

How did your body feel after today's shift?

_____
_____
_____
_____

What's one thing you want to reset or release?

_____
_____
_____
_____

How can you support yourself before your next shift?

_____
_____
_____
_____
_____

You've been on alert all day. It's time to rest without guilt.

DAY 82

What's something that challenged you today?

_____

_____

_____

_____

_____

What's something that gave you joy or purpose?

_____

_____

_____

_____

_____

How did your body feel after today's shift?

_____

_____

_____

_____

_____

What's one thing you want to reset or release?

_____

_____

_____

_____

_____

How can you support yourself before your next shift?

_____

_____

_____

_____

_____

Don't skip meals. You can't pour from an empty stomach either.

DAY 83

What's something that challenged you today?

_____

_____

_____

_____

_____

What's something that gave you joy or purpose?

_____

_____

_____

_____

_____

How did your body feel after today's shift?

_____

_____

_____

_____

_____

What's one thing you want to reset or release?

_____

_____

_____

_____

_____

How can you support yourself before your next shift?

_____

_____

_____

_____

_____

Silence is a strategy. Use it to return to yourself.

DAY 84

What's something that challenged you today?

_____

_____

_____

_____

_____

What's something that gave you joy or purpose?

_____

_____

_____

_____

_____

How did your body feel after today's shift?

_____

_____

_____

_____

_____

What's one thing you want to reset or release?

_____

_____

_____

_____

_____

How can you support yourself before your next shift?

_____

_____

_____

_____

_____

Your worth isn't tied to your productivity. You're already enough.

DAY 85

What's something that challenged you today?

_____

_____

_____

_____

_____

What's something that gave you joy or purpose?

_____

_____

_____

_____

_____

How did your body feel after today's shift?

_____

_____

_____

_____

What's one thing you want to reset or release?

_____

_____

_____

_____

How can you support yourself before your next shift?

_____

_____

_____

_____

_____

A cold drink. A quiet room. A slow exhale. Reset the moment.

DAY 86

What's something that challenged you today?

_____

_____

_____

_____

_____

What's something that gave you joy or purpose?

_____

_____

_____

_____

_____

How did your body feel after today's shift?

_____

_____

_____

_____

_____

What's one thing you want to reset or release?

_____

_____

_____

_____

_____

How can you support yourself before your next shift?

_____

_____

_____

_____

_____

You're not lazy. You're depleted. That's not the
same thing.

DAY 87

What's something that challenged you today?

_____

_____

_____

_____

_____

What's something that gave you joy or purpose?

_____

_____

_____

_____

_____

How did your body feel after today's shift?

_____

_____

_____

_____

_____

What's one thing you want to reset or release?

_____

_____

_____

_____

_____

How can you support yourself before your next shift?

_____

_____

_____

_____

Light stretching. Minimal scrolling. Let your mind and body recalibrate.

DAY 88

What's something that challenged you today?

_____
_____
_____
_____
_____

What's something that gave you joy or purpose?

_____
_____
_____
_____
_____

How did your body feel after today's shift?

_____
_____
_____
_____
_____

What's one thing you want to reset or release?

_____
_____
_____
_____
_____

How can you support yourself before your next shift?

_____
_____
_____
_____
_____

Burnout doesn't ask permission. Catch it before it catches you.

DAY 89

What's something that challenged you today?

_____

_____

_____

_____

_____

What's something that gave you joy or purpose?

_____

_____

_____

_____

_____

How did your body feel after today's shift?

_____

_____

_____

_____

_____

What's one thing you want to reset or release?

_____

_____

_____

_____

_____

How can you support yourself before your next shift?

_____

_____

_____

_____

_____

Gentle foods. Soft music. Eye mask. You deserve comfort, not just survival.

DAY 90

What's something that challenged you today?

_____

_____

_____

_____

_____

What's something that gave you joy or purpose?

_____

_____

_____

_____

_____

How did your body feel after today's shift?

_____

_____

_____

_____

_____

What's one thing you want to reset or release?

_____

_____

_____

_____

_____

How can you support yourself before your next shift?

_____

_____

_____

_____

_____

You made it to Day 90. That's not just progress --
that's power.

You've made it through the heavy days --
now carry forward with lighter steps,
stronger purpose, and unshakable self-worth.
Keep going. You're not done growing.
I'm proud of you.
- Cel Robinson, BSN RN

FROM ONE SHIFT TO ANOTHER...

Thank you for allowing this journal to be part of your journey.
Whether you filled every page or simply paused to breathe, you did
something powerful:

you showed up for yourself.

In the moments between chaos and calm, I hope you found a space to
reconnect —
not just with your role, but with your heart.

Keep resetting.
Keep healing.

You're never alone in this.
Imacel ·Cel· Robinson, BSN RN

@officiallookitscelly